LOSING WEIGHT

Making A Complete Lifestyle Change

Lisa Heskett

Table of Contents

Introduction

Congratulations on downloading *Losing Weight: Making A Complete Lifestyle Change* and thank you for doing so. If you truly want to lose weight and keep it off, changing your entire life perspective is the only way to do so. This book is the first step to finding the motivation, planning and executing your lifestyle change!

The following chapters will discuss how to shed pounds and keep it off—the right way. The world of weight loss doesn't have to be scary and riddled with fad diets and failure. This book is here to help you make the real lifestyle changes needed to lose weight and keep it off.

For starters, you will learn how to find motivation and set proper goals for your health quest. Knowing how to set a S.M.A.R.T. goal can make or break your success! You will also learn about basic nutrition, and how to eat properly for weight loss. Prepare to conquer smoothies, meal prepping, and freezer bag meals! You'll find tips and tricks that go above and beyond the normal diet that will help yours stick for good.

Exercise is also hugely important in weight loss, and this book does not neglect ideas for simple at home workouts! There are workouts for every muscle in your body, all that you can do without purchasing a single piece of workout equipment. There are also tips for preventing injury, and how to build your body up at a comfortable pace so you never get wary of working out. If you needed any more convincing, check out the short and long-term affects a healthier lifestyle has on your body as well!

There are plenty of books on this subject on the market, thanks again for choosing this one! Every effort was made to ensure it is full of as much useful information as possible, please enjoy!

Chapter 1

Understanding a Healthy Lifestyle

The first step to losing weight and building yourself a healthier life is to get a plan ready and to get organized! Making the necessary changes to take charge of your health and lose weight can be daunting, but not so much with proper planning and execution. Understanding how nutrition and exercise fit into weight loss are important as well, so you are able to accurately plan and make informed decisions.

Finding Motivation to Get Started

Buying this book shows that you have the startup motivation needed to make a lifestyle change! If you want your switch to stick however, you'll need more than a quick burst of inspiration.

Begin by thinking of the *why*—why are you thinking of losing weight in the first place? Should weight loss or muscle toning be the goal? Do you want to go up stairs lightning quick or is your focus on feeling more confident in your clothing? Write out your goals, no matter how silly or small they may seem. Try to think of long-term and short-term goals with specific time limits (but don't hold yourself too harshly on them, more on that later). Keep this all in a Fitness Journal, and look back on it if you ever forget *why* you're working so hard!

Setting Realistic Goals

When you're beginning to make lifestyle changes, realistic goal setting is crucial. You may remember S.M.A.R.T. goals, which were a popular lesson in many schools due to its accuracy! The acronym may have stood for slightly different things, but the general ideas for S.M.A.R.T. goals were:

- Specific—a goal should very clearly define what you hope to accomplish *lose 50 lbs*

- Measurable—keep goals quantifiable, for example "I want to lose weight," vs. "I want to lose 15 pounds."

- Action-Oriented—be sure to include how exactly you plan to achieve your goal, what specific steps are required to finish to complete goal

- Realistic—this may seem like common sense, but it can be very easy to get carried away with your goals and make them too unattainable, thus allowing you to get discouraged when you don't reach your goals by the time set and possibly creating further setbacks

- Time-Based—make sure this is a reasonable (and for our purposes healthy) amount of time to fully complete your goal; however, don't allow too much time and accidentally inhibit your improvement *8 months or more.*

Your goals should be healthy for your body. If you want to truly lose weight and keep it off, it will be a slow uphill battle, with occasional dips and times you'll want to quit. If you expect progress too fast, you will eventually not be able to reach your goals and become discouraged. Don't add extra obstacles for yourself, plan your goals carefully.

2

Support Systems

While of course you can do this on your own, having the right support system can really make or break a weight loss program! If possible, try to find someone who has similar goals as you and work on them together. Two is always better than one, and having someone who understands what you are undergoing can be such a relief! An added benefit of having a partner-in-crime (or several) is that you can always hold each other accountable. Accountability is one thing that is easy to start being lax after the first few weeks of a new weight loss program, especially if results aren't quite where you want them to be.

Never Underestimate #Fitspo

Similar to support groups, never underestimate the power of a little bit of fitness inspiration! Check out different hashtags on Instagram, Pinterest, Facebook, Twitter, or Tumblr for inspiration from the millions of others who are undertaking the same journey as you! Just like reviewing at your goals, browsing some of the inspirational fitness posts out there can help refocus you! Check out pictures, look at pictures of healthy and delicious food. Also, these websites are fantastic if you want some more ideas for what exercises to do on what days. There are plenty of fun, quick little exercises out there that "Burn 100 calories"—add these up over the course of your day and you have knocked off 500 calories (where that number comes from below)! While you're reaching your goals, make sure to put out some #fitspo of your own!

Losing Pounds: How It Works

Losing weight can be represented as an actual mathematical equation.

$$1 \ lb = 3,500 \ calories$$

This means that in order to lose one pound of body fat, you're going to need to find a way to get rid of 3,500 calories. Sounds daunting at first, but it's not so bad if you break if it up over the course of the week!

3,500 cal/7 days in week = 500 calories per day

If you want to lose a single pound in one week, you could do so by shaving 500 calories a day. A common rule of thumb for weight loss says that success relies on 80 percent diet, 20 percent exercise. This holds true because it is easier to cut out some calories via intake than it is to burn them via exercise (which is still important for a healthy lifestyle). You may notice that in the early on, a few more pounds are shedding off each week. Once you've got a routine down, a healthy amount of weight to lose is only one to two pounds per week.

While exercise is less efficient when it comes to eliminating a quota of calories, it is still crucial to a happier, healthier life. The benefits of exercise are never ending; don't cheat yourself out of them.

Keep in mind that as you are keeping track of your progress, your weight will fluctuate and sometimes it is better to lose inches than pounds. Muscle weighs more than fat, so don't be discouraged if you're not seeing the specific number on the scale you're hoping for. Be patient, and trust that you have decided to lose weight the right way!

Note: You may want to visit your doctor before you begin any extreme diet or exercise changes. You should get a yearly physical done and regularly talk with your doctor about your health goals— they may even be able to offer some invaluable advice that you wouldn't have found anywhere else!

Chapter 2

Diet & Nutrition: The First 80%

It's been established that diet is the largest factor in weight loss—you can lose weight without exercise but not so much the other way around. We're all familiar with the food pyramid, but who actually refers to it when making meal decisions for the day? And counting calories can be a drag. Going on a diet doesn't have to mean misery—it just means being a bit more thoughtful about what you're consuming.

For the best results with your dietary changes, try to keep things simple. But first, take this opportunity and clean out your pantry! Out with the old, in with the new. Plus, it's best to put yourself as far from temptation as possible.

Now it's time to start your grocery list. Whether you are planning on cooking throughout the week or you want to begin meal prepping (more on recipes and meal prep next chapter) What kinds of foods should be on your list if you're trying to lose weight?

Meats/Proteins

Proteins are essential to your body for building and repairing processes. This is why protein shakes are so popular, and vegetarians/vegans face so many dietary problems. The recommended amount of protein per day is 46 grams for women and 56 grams for men, which ends up being a pretty small budget if you're a hard-core meat eater (an 8 oz. steak has around 50 grams of protein!). Keep protein lean to avoid high cholesterol, and as much as you may want to, try not to eat red meat as your entire daily protein. Keep in mind that most dairy products offer protein also, as well as the much-needed Vitamin D! Here are some healthy options to get your daily protein, pick a few and add to your shopping list:

- Lean cuts of steak

- 95% Ground Beef—or better yet, replace with ground turkey (season it well and no one will notice!)

- Boneless, skinless chicken breasts

- Light Tuna

- Salmon

- Tilapia

- Dried lentils

- Sandwich meat—roasted turkey or roast beef

- Turkey Jerky

- Mixed nuts/peanuts

- Protein powder (for smoothies)

- Quinoa

- Greek Yogurt

- Milk

- Cottage Cheese

- Eggs

Fruits & Veggies

Fruits and vegetables are packed with the vitamins and nutrients you need to look and feel great (and the fiber will help keep you full for longer). Not only are fruits and vegetables great for your diet, they're also great for your wallet. Produce can be shopped seasonally to save money, or go out and support your local farmers' market. Five servings of each are recommended a day. That's a lot of food! Vegetables make for great sides and fruits are perfect for a sweet treat after dinner (drizzle some honey over a fruit bowl with a dollop of Greek yogurt—yum). When buying fruits and vegetables, a good rule of thumb is to keep your cart colorful. Here are some ideas of fruits and vegetables to add to your shopping list:

- *Vegetables:* cucumbers, spinach, romaine lettuce, bell peppers (all colors, red bell peppers are especially linked to weight loss), tomatoes, onions, kale, broccoli, Brussels sprouts, peas, carrots, asparagus, okra, scallions, green beans, cauliflower, avocado, zucchini, squash, celery, corn, potatoes, sweet potatoes

- *Fruits:* apples, bananas, strawberries, grapefruit, blackberries, blueberries, mangoes, papayas, cherries, cranberries, grapes, kiwis, oranges, peaches, pears, pineapples, watermelon, pomegranates

Carbs—The Good Kind

Carbs can be scary, because no one can seem to really agree on them. Dietary guidelines, however, suggest that carbs take up half our daily caloric intake. The point of carbohydrates is to provide us with energy, but it also easily stored as fat. Carbohydrates and fiber come hand in hand.

It is important to understand the distinction between a good and a bad carb, or a "whole" carb and a "refined" carb. Generally speaking, a refined carb is going to be very processed and likely have a bunch of sugar mixed in. You can find whole carbs in fruit, vegetables, sweet potatoes, regular potatoes, and legumes. Wheat pasta and bread can also supply healthy carbohydrates. Any carb with the word "white" in front of it you may want to avoid: white pasta, white rice, and white bread.

Healthy Snacks

Since you tossed out your junk food, make sure to replace it with easy grab and go snacks that will satisfy your craving without taking too much out of your daily calories. Make your own trail mix with assorted nuts, pretzels, and dark chocolate! When picking snacks, include some options that are a little extra salty or a little extra sweet without over doing it—it's nice to have something to grab when an extreme craving hits that you don't have to feel bad about. Eating snacks throughout the day will also help you not overeat at regular meals. Some more snack ideas (so you can add things to your list as needed):

- Assorted fruit—Fruit ends up being the toughest food group to fit into your day. Solve this by having the fruit around your house for a snack! It'll help curb the craving for sweets as well since fruits are packed with natural sugars.

- Nuts—The protein helps curb hunger pangs, but be wary of over-eating nuts (they can be pretty high in fat and caloric content). Stick with unsalted to prevent bloating.

- Granola bars/other prepackaged "healthy" snacks—Use caution and read the labels. Some of these aren't half bad, just make sure you aren't eating a bar loaded down with corn syrup. However, if you do find the right bar they are a great grab-and-go option if you are in a hurry.

- Chips & Salsa—filling and low calorie, as long as you stay away from chips that are too salty this is a great snack!

- Uncooked Veggies—Celery with peanut butter, carrots with ranch, and fresh bell peppers. Vegetables are high in fiber and low in sugar, keeping you fuller longer. This will also help you get your recommended serving of vegetables for the day.

- Hardboiled eggs—sprinkle a little pepper and mustard on this tasty appetite busting snack.

Cheat Well, Cheat (Semi) Often

You will never stick to making a healthy lifestyle change if you expect yourself to quit all of your favorite foods in an instant. Allow yourself a cheat meal a week, and move on and be done with it. Just make sure that your cheat meal stays within reason—don't eat an entire pepperoni pizza with extra sausage just because it's your cheat day. Keep in mind portion control and never forget what you're working for. Give your taste buds a chance to adjust (while allowing several cheats), and soon you will prefer the more wholesome food.

And even if you end up slipping up and having a cheat meal turn into, say a cheat week, don't think it's ever too late to get back on the horse. Sometimes life happens, and unfortunately your diet and exercise (two of the things that can help you mentally and emotionally tackle obstacles, ironically enough) end up taking the hit. It's okay—just push forward.

Yes, Have a Sip

When drinking an alcoholic beverage, keep in mind how many calories are in what you're sipping. Is it worth wrecking your health goals? That's not to say you can't successfully have a healthy lifestyle and regularly consume alcohol, but never forget that moderation is key. Try switching to alcoholic drinks that are lighter in calories or have a glass of red wine (which has been linked to cardiovascular health). Stick to lighter alcohols with simple mixers to enjoy a buzz without having feel guilty about it, not that you should anyways. As far as sugary sodas go, it's best to just stay away altogether. In summary, don't waste your calories on drinks!

Chapter 3

Put Your Plan Into Action

Now that you are fully aware of the types of food you should eating, let's look at how some basic meal planning can change your life!

When you're trying to lose weight, you will hear over and over that it is the little things. This is true! There are some swaps that you can make that will go undetectable, and save a ton of calories/fat/sugar/bad things in the process:

- Almond or coconut milk for your 2 percent. Don't worry; we're not suggesting you stop buying your favorite milk. Just buy some almond milk and sneak it in places in lieu of milk where you won't notice it, like cereal or swap for half of your creamer in your coffee.

- Greek Yogurt—it may require a taste bud adjustment, so start off with the vanilla if you're not already a yogurt lover. Swap plain Greek yogurt for sour cream on chicken chili (recipe below). Put berries on vanilla yogurt and have a parfait for breakfast that is packed with nutrients and probiotics!

- Quinoa and brown rice for white rice—with proper seasoning, it's guaranteed you won't miss your plain old white rice. And you shouldn't be buying white bread for any reason.

- Buy the light version of your favorite products. The light ranch, the light butter, so on and so forth. It's going to taste different at first, but before long your taste buds will adapt (and you will probably end up preferring the light version).

One way that's become increasingly popular to diet is to meal prep, and this is actually a great tool at your disposal to really make a lifestyle change! With meal prepping, you can control what you are eating and always have food ready on hand, thus preventing you from just getting drive thru on the way home.

Meal Prep—The How

Preparing your meals for an *entire week* is a concept that can be overwhelming and exciting. You still have to do the work, but you're doing it all at once (Sundays are a popular meal prep day) so it's ready to go when you need it through the week. This can also help you save money if you properly plan and execute! When you're first getting started, there are some things to keep in mind:

- The containers you're going to use—you may have a full stock of Tupperware, or you may need to stock up a little bit. Ideally, you want containers that are all the same and stackable. The containers should be clear as well so you can see what's inside easily, and it's worth buying some labels if you want to keep your fridge even more organized. Make sure they're also BPA free, dishwasher safe, and microwaveable!

- Break the cooking into two or more days. Prepare all the ingredients you will need (cut the vegetables, portion out whatever you need specifically for recipes, etc.), but don't do all of your cooking in one day—you'll get extremely overwhelmed and might even want to quit. Do a bulk cooking on Sunday and a refresher on Wednesday, whatever works best for you.

- Decide where meal prepping will help your life the most, and make that a focus! If you're regularly not eating breakfast and your excuse is that there's nothing ready for you to eat besides cereal, make some breakfast burritos!

- Incorporate things that don't require cooking also—make sandwiches ready to go (just don't put the condiments on the bread) or an oatmeal bag that's just-add-water!

- Not every meal that you prepare has to be uber healthy. It's okay to throw in some of your old favorites—just make some of the healthy switches previously mentioned in your recipes and remember balance.

- Don't try all new recipes the first time. It'll make things take that much longer, and make you not want to try again. Do print off the new recipes you are using—when you're cooking and your hands are dirty, you're not going to want to stop constantly to check your phone or computer.

- Know that meal prep takes some practice to find what's best for you and your household. Don't get discouraged and keep notes each time so you don't forget things you want to try next time.

- Meal prepping doesn't have to be a recipe ordeal all the time either. Don't fret too much if you don't have a specific recipe lined out—grill some meat and vegetables and throw it in container with quinoa and viola, lunch is done.

Shakes & Smoothies

If you don't have a blender, it's time to go purchase one. They come at a variety of prices and qualities—you don't have to break the bank for your first one! Once you know the basics of crafting a good shake and see the results, you'll wonder how you ever lived without one! To build a shake, follow these guidelines: 1 cup greens, 1 cup fruit, and 1 cup liquid. Many recipes vary from this model, but it's a good place to start. Put the liquid in your blender first, as it will help your blender work better because the blades are wet. Start on the lowest setting until bigger chunks are broke up, and don't worry if your drink is too runny—just add a few ice cubes and problem solved.

Shakes and smoothies are a great way to get your servings in as well as some protein if you use protein powder! With protein powder, you can replace a full meal. Prep smoothies ahead by portioning out your greens (a mix of spinach and kale is best) and your fruits separately into bags. In most major grocery stores, there are also a variety of frozen fruits already cut, just put them in a Ziploc baggie and you are good! If you're wanting to use protein powder, start with the vanilla flavor and keep in mind that it may be pricey but does last for quite a while assuming you follow the instructions and only use in smoothies meant to be meal replacements.

Test out some of these smoothies and shakes and enjoy:

- Green Strawanna—combine 1 cup greens, ½ cup frozen strawberries ½ cup frozen strawberries, and one cup milk product. A classic made even better! Add protein powder and this is a great breakfast.

- Mango & Lime—combine ¾ frozen mango, ½ cup green grapes, 1 cup greens, ½ cup water, and a tablespoon of fresh lime juice. Sweet with the perfect bit of sour.

- Iced Coffee Protein Shake—combine 1 cup cold coffee, ¾ cups milk product, 2 cups (or heaping handfuls) off ice, and a scoop of protein powder (vanilla or chocolate). A nice, filling pick me up! If you want it to be a little sweeter, add some honey or cocoa powder.

- Chocolate Peanut Butter—combine 1 tablespoon peanut butter, 1 cup milk product, 1 tablespoon cocoa powder, 1 scoop protein powder (or another tablespoon of peanut butter), a handful of ice, 1 tablespoon honey, and a pinch of cinnamon.

The beauty of shakes and smoothies are that they are completely customizable. Replace some of your liquid with a dollop of Greek Yogurt to give it a little extra oomph, or add some chai or flax seeds. This is also a great place to use that milk replacement!

Get Cooking

Eating at home not only saves you money, it saves you calories. Unfortunately, this means you're going to have to do the cooking yourself. Luckily for you, there are so many more resources available now to newbie chefs than there were in any other time period, all thanks to the good ole' Internet. And keep in mind that not every meal you make at home has to be perfectly healthy. It's okay to splurge as long as your keep your head with portion control.

But for now, try out some of the recipes below that are so easy anyone can do them, but so amazingly tasty that you'll be blown away that you actually get to eat this stuff on your "diet".

Five Ingredient Chicken Chili

Serves 6

What You'll Need...

- 6 c. chicken broth

- 1 jar salsa verde (2 cups worth)

- 4 cups fully cooked shredded chicken (can used canned or shred yourself)

- 2 (15 oz.) cans Great Northern beans, rinsed & drained

- Pinch of cumin

- *Topping Ideas*: shredded low fat cheese, diced avocado, cilantro, chopped green onions, plain Greek yogurt, crumbled tortilla chips

Combine in a large pot over medium high, bring to a boil and turn back down. Cook as long as you like, or put in your crockpot!

Chicken Fajita Bowls

Serves 4

What You'll Need...

- 2-3 grilled chicken breast, sliced

- 1 can whole kernel corn

- ¾ cup quinoa

- Lime

- 2 bell peppers (any color)

- Salt and pepper to taste

Lightly sauté vegetables together in olive oil, then cook corn and quinoa separate (add a dash of cumin in the quinoa). Keep the quinoa and vegetables separate in the container, refrigerate or freeze.

Frozen Breakfast Burritos

8 Servings

What You'll Need...

- 2 cups cooked tater tots

- ½ pound meat (sausage, bacon, or omit entirely for vegetarian option)

- Any vegetables you want to add—tomatoes, onions, and bell peppers work great

- 1/3 cup milk (can split with almond milk to make a little healthier)

- 8 large eggs lightly beaten

- 1 (16-ounce) can refried beans

- 8 (8-inch) wheat flour tortillas

- 2 cups low fat shredded cheese

- Salt and pepper to taste

Heat some olive oil in a large skillet over medium high heat. Prepare your meat/vegetables of choice and use a little of the remainder liquid fat to cook the eggs. Spread the refried beans on the tortillas—this really gives your morning breakfast burrito a little something extra!

Build burrito with meat/vegetables, eggs, cheeses, and any other extras you can think of. To freeze the burritos, cover each one tightly with aluminum foil. Keeps for a month in the freezer. To heat, bake at 450 degrees F for twenty minutes, (microwave for 5-6 minutes) or until completely cooked through.

One Pan Salmon & Veggies

4 Servings

What You'll Need...

- 4 salmon filets

- 1-2 large sweet potatoes, cut into strips or diced

- 1 bunch asparagus

- Olive oil

- Salt and pepper

- 1 lemon

Set the oven to 425 degrees F. Lightly coat the potatoes in olive oil, sprinkle with salt and pepper (if you like a dash of spice, add a dash of paprika or chili powder). Spread the sweet potatoes evenly on a pre greased pan (line with aluminum to save time on cleanup), and bake for 20 minutes, or until the potatoes are just about cooked. Remove from oven and carefully scoot all of the sweet potatoes to one side of the pan, stack them up if need to be evenly spread out the salmon and asparagus on the pan. Lightly drizzle olive oil on the salmon and asparagus, and finish with lemon juice. Cook about 10 more minutes! This recipe would be great for midweek with having all of the vegetables cut and ready to go, or as a family meal! Use the cold left over salmon to add protein to your salad.

Two Ingredient Banana Pancakes

4 Servings

What You'll Need...

- 2 ripe bananas

- 2 large eggs

Using a fork, mash the banana in an appropriately sized mixing bowl. Mash it into the consistency of pudding with few-to-no lumps, and then lightly whisk in any of the powder extras mentioned below. In a separate bowl, whisk eggs until they are completely smooth and then pour over the bananas. Once you've finished your batter (which will be much more liquidy than normal pancake batter, but never fear), you're ready for a hot skillet. Don't forget to lightly grease the pan so it doesn't stick, and when you're ready drop about two tablespoons of the mixture in the skillet, and you should hear a sizzle right away. Softly sprinkle your chunkier additional toppings now, and let cook for one minute. Flip the pancakes gently—the center will still be a bit jiggly. In fact, some of the batter might spill out a little. This is fine! Use the spatula to lightly nudge your pancake back over the spill, and cook for another minute. Pancake sides should be golden brown, and it'll be much more solid! Top with syrup, jam, honey, or some lite whipped cream.

There are some other things you can add to your pancakes to alter the flavor and texture just a tad: a pinch of baking powder (to make them fluffier), salt, cinnamon, vanilla, cocoa powder, honey, dark chocolate, granola, or fruit! You can refrigerate or freeze these pancakes as well for a tasty quick breakfast or snack.

Salads

If you're trying to lose weight, you're going to want to eat a salad at some point in time. Salads don't have to be boring or a drag though! For a weeks' worth of salad, here's what you will need:

- Large container of base greens—you can switch this up by using spinach, romaine, or mixing some kale in

- Package cherry tomatoes

- 2 cucumbers

- 1 avocado

- 2 bell peppers

- 5 carrots

- 1 can chickpeas

- Sunflower seeds

- Your favorite dressing—lean towards oil based dressings, and check the labels for high sugar, sodium, or calories.

To pack salads for work, you'll need a solution for dressing. Some people like the "Mason Jar Salads" which actually work great because the dressing is at the bottom, far away from your lettuce. Alternatively, you can purchase plastic ramekins that are a perfect portion of dressing and some companies have reusable to go ramekins in their bundles!

Freezer Bag & Crock Pot Meals

You should definitely consider adding some of the popular "freezer bag" meals into you weekly meal prep! Usually they require no cooking and are cost efficient. Some of the recipes found on the Internet can be high in sodium or fat however, so just be cautious (or don't, because not every single meal you make has to be uber healthy). You're still making your week easier by making them ahead. Most of them you can simply dump in the crockpot before work, pop it on low and enjoy the benefits of a homemade meal at ridiculously low effort. Use that time to squeeze in a quick workout!

When making your freezer bag meals, be sure to label the bags clearly with full information: how long it needs to cook, what temperature, and anything you need to add to the bag's contents once it's in your slow cooker. It also never hurts to double bag, and you can thaw the night before if you desire (not strictly necessary but it definitely makes getting it in the slow cooker a little easier).

Try out some of these recipes:

Turkey Sloppy Joes

4-6 Servings

High for 3-4 hours

What You'll Need...

- 1 lb ground turkey

- 1 diced onion

- 1 diced green bell pepper

- 15 oz. can tomato sauce

- Sloppy Joe seasoning packet

Cranberry Pork

6 servings

Low for 8-10 hours

What You'll Need...

- 2-3 pounds pork roast

- 2 cups fresh or frozen cranberries

- ½ cup orange juice concentrate

- 1 tablespoon brown or Dijon mustard

- 1 onion, dice

- Salt & pepper

- ¼ teaspoon ground cinnamon

Beef and Vegetable Stew

6 servings

Low for 8 hours, add the beef broth

What You'll Need...

- 2 lbs beef chuck roast

- 2 celery ribs chopped

- 3 carrots, peeled and chopped

- 1/2 onion chopped

- 1 bay leaf

- 2 tsp dried thyme

- 1 tsp dried rosemary

- 1/2 tsp salt

- 1/4 tsp ground black pepper

- 1/2 cup pearled barley

- 7 cups beef broth (day of cooking)

Ranch Shredded Chicken Tacos

6 servings

Low for 6-8 hours

What You'll Need...

- 2 lbs boneless skinless chicken breasts

- 3 tablespoons olive oil

- 2 tablespoons red wine vinegar

- 1 tablespoon chili powder

- Salt and pepper to taste

- ½ tsp of each of ground paprika cumin, garlic powder, red pepper flakes, oregano, and onion powder

- 1 dry ranch seasoning packet, try spicy for a little extra kick

Chapter 4

Get Ready To Move

While diet and nutrition make up the majority of weight loss, you still can't forget the other twenty percent! Making the steps to have an active lifestyle will help you really push to the results you are seeking! Furthermore, exercising regularly will help you push past the inevitable weight loss "plateau", as well as provide so many other long term health benefits. A gym membership isn't necessary to reap the benefits from exercise—all of the workouts listed in this book are ones you can do from the comfort of your own home.

Know Your Body's Limits (& Respect Them)

When starting a new exercise plan, first take a look at your current fitness level. Could you comfortable run a mile? Can you go up the stairs without feeling winded? If not, no worries—you'll get there! Through slow training and plenty of stretching, you can effectively use exercise to reach your health goals.

The suggested amount of exercise from the U.S. Department of Health is about 30 minutes of moderate activity five times a week (or a total of 150 minutes spaced out in any way). Look at your schedule for the week, and see where you can squeeze in a quick exercise.

Don't forget to allow plenty of time for recovery—especially in the beginning, because you're going to be sore. To combat overworking your muscles, make sure to rotate muscle areas that you are going to working on and take a day off every now and then!

Finally, it is crucial that you always have proper equipment and apparel to prevent injuries. Find the proper tennis shoes that fit right, have the proper clothing and use the right equipment for your strength level.

Move More!

It's time to take notice of your daily step count. Generally, the daily step count recommendation is around 10,000 steps. Unless you work a job that requires you to move around a lot, this can be quite a feat! The key is to try to sneak extra steps in every way that you can. Here are some ideas to incorporate in your every day life:

- Use the time that you would spend driving around the parking lot smarter—instead, park your car farther away from the door, forcing you to walk more! Use the parking trick anywhere—work, restaurants, school, etc.

- Take the stairs, and keep on your tiptoes! You may feel the burn, but it's a great workout for your calves!

- Take the dog for quick walk around the block—Fido will be grateful for the exercise too.

- Walk and talk. When you're talking on the phone in your home, pace your hall, kitchen, living room, and bedroom. Walk all over the house; maybe add a hop or a skip!

- If you work a desk job, try to take frequent walks. Be it the bathroom, the coffee pot, or the break room, try to take a quick five minute walk when you can.

- Have some fun window-shopping! Malls are great places to walk long distances and enjoy the benefits of being indoors. Malls even tend to open their doors a little early for walkers. If you are actually shopping, pace the full distance of the mall before your first purchase.

- Treat yourself to your favorite television program, but walk through the commercials.

- Skip the drive thru. Get the extra steps, and it sometimes ends up being faster than waiting in line!

- Housework and yard work are a great way to get steps, and get your house cleaned. It's a win-win, even if it's not the most fun. As the famous slogan goes, just do it.

Basically, you should take any opportunity to walk instead of be still. If you are sitting for an extended period of time, break it up with short walks or at least stretch. By all means, rest when you're tired but listen to your body—are your legs feeling restless? That means it's time get up!

Using a pedometer to count your steps can help you keep on track. You can get a low-tech pedometer for cheap for invest in one of the many wrist fitness-trackers on the market (i.e., Fitbit, Garmin, Misfit and more). These and smart watches can give you so much more information than just steps, such as your resting heart rate, active minutes, and sleep patterns.

Walking Versus Running

There are a plethora of opinions out there on the subject of weight loss in regards to walking versus running. What it really boils down to: both are great for cardiovascular health and weight loss, so try to incorporate whichever you're actually comfortable with the most.

Mile for mile, running burns more calories (due to the fact it simply takes more energy). Therefore, running is going to burn more fat off of your body and make you thinner quicker. Running has also recently been shown to actually suppress your appetite, ensuring you don't eat back all of the calories you just burned! If you only have a short time to work out and are really wanting to get your heart rate up, a quick jog is a great way.

On the flip side of the coin, walking tends to provide better long-term health benefits than solely running—between a group of people who walk and run the same amount of time, the walkers would have a further reduced risk of heart disease and high cholesterol than the runners.

In summary, when starting out your new workout program, include a mix of walking and running that will work for you. If you're new to running, start in small increments and slowly build up your time. And never forget, the first few workouts are always the hardest!

OMMM

Yoga has become one of the more popular exercise programs in the last decade, and with good reason. It's simple, feels great, and has some amazing side effects on the mind and body! Yoga isn't a particularly high calorie burner (only about 150 calories an hour, in comparison to 300 from walking), but it's a great addition to your weight loss program for a multitude of reasons!

For one, it'll help alleviate some of the soreness you're experiencing from the rest of your exercise routine! The stretches are great to remember for even immediately after a workout to help your muscles cool down. Many poses are designed to build strength, which can help your other workouts!

Yoga is also good for your mental health. It can be looked at as a type of meditation—you're focusing on your breathing and body, listening to your muscles and joints, and getting in tune with your 'self''.

Gyms & Classes

Some people find that actually paying for a gym membership or a specific class helps them find the motivation to get their workout in. This may or may not be the best solution to building a healthier life for yourself, but it's definitely worth the consideration! Most gym sign ups also include at least one free session with a personal trainer, which can be useful even one time to get some tips for your fitness goals!

Classes can be great because there are groups designed for different interests and varying skill levels. Some classes make it seem more like a fun dance session than a work out, such as Zumba and Jazzercise. There are plenty of other types of classes to try, like kickboxing, yoga (or hot yoga for the braver heart), cycling and more!

The most important factor of an exercise program is making sure it's one you're actually going to follow. It's easy to give up or get discouraged when you miss a workout (or a weeks' worth), but always be willing to make adjustments and forgive yourself! It's always going to be alright if you are willing to make the steps to get back on track.

Chapter 5

Work Every Muscle

The first step to a full workout is elevating your heart rate to get your body in prime calorie burning mode. Go for a brisk walk or jog, do some jumping jacks, or dance around to your favorite song!

Once you've got your heart rate up, it's time to get some strength training done. Having an overall toned body increases your metabolic rate, thus strength workouts need to be a part of every exercise program. Again, it is crucial to rotate which section of your body you work on so as to not create injuries and put a hold on your progress!

Arms, Shoulders, & Back

As far as starting a new workout program goes, upper body strength is usually not anyone's strong suit right off the bat (unless your job requires lifting of some kind). This being said, take your build up slow. Here are some exercises you can do around the house (minimal equipment) to help build your upper body strength:

- Pushups ("girl" pushups on your knees will work)—Try them with your feet on an exercise ball for some extra challenge. 10 - 20 reps is a good starting amount and work your way up

- Arm Raises—Stand with your feet shoulder-width apart, and with weights (canned goods will do if you haven't purchased weights yet) slowly raise your arms in front of you, then to the side and back to start position. Fifteen or so reps are a good place to start.

- Bench Dips—For this you'll need to sturdy surfaces that can support your full body weight: two chairs, a chair and a medicine ball, anything about two feet off the ground. Hold your body up using your arms and legs, and use your arms to dip your body so you are parallel to the floor. This one can be a bit more demanding on your joints, so start small (around 10 reps or so).

- Arm curls—With your weights or cans, start with your arms at a 90 degree angle in front of you, palms up. Bending your elbows, bring your hands up to your chin and back down for one rep. Depending on the amount of weight you're using, start off with 15-25 reps.

Core/Abdominal

The core is the popular target of many people beginning their exercise program, and for good reason! A strong core is the building block for a stronger body—it can help you lift, push the extra distance, and keep your back strong from injuries. Try to incorporate some of these abdominal workouts into your new program!

- Crunches/sit-ups—The most common exercise for your abdomen for it's simplicity and ability to be customized. Use proper form when doing crunches: if it hurts your back or spine, something is not quite right and you are definitely doing more harm than good. For basic crunches, begin on your back, knees slightly bent and hands behind your head. Open your elbows wide, and lift your shoulders up about nine inches from the ground (exhale as you lift). Keep you neck movement natural, meaning don't strain up or tuck down. For the best

31

results, crunches should also be a more deliberate process, not a speed test. You can alternate crunches by adding a twist with your knees/elbows, or stick your feet straight in the air attempt a reverse crunch.

- Posture holding—When you're in a plank position, ten seconds can feel like thirty minutes. Holding tough resistance postures greatly accelerate your core strength. To perform a simple plank, begin on your stomach and lift up using only your forearms and toes. Your body should run in a straight line in this position. After some practice, try side planks (only rotate your body to be facing the wall rather than the floor, body weight on one arm perpendicular to your body). When you're done with planks, roll on your belly and try a Superman: lie flat with arms overhead and legs straight. Lift your arms and legs as high as you can off the ground, and hold the position with your abs held tight for five to ten seconds.

- Birddog—Start evenly distributed on your hands and knees and your back flat. Extend straight (keep parallel to the floor) your right arm and left leg, and hold the posture for five seconds. This takes some serious practice and balance! Start with eight-ten reps per alternate side.

- Bridge—A great position to hold at the end of your exercise. Start on your back, legs straight but knees relaxed with arms at your side. Pull your feet up to a comfortable position to lift your lower back off the ground using your abdominal muscles and glutes. If you hold the position properly and practice deep breathing, this will end up feeling like more of a stretch!

- Speaking of stretching, don't forget about your abdominals. Start on your stomach and using your hands (palms flat on the floor) slowly roll your head/neck/spine. Yes, you will look like a seal, and it will feel amazing once your arms are fully straightened.

Legs & Glutes

Some of your largest and strongest muscles reside in your legs. Treat them well, and you will find that you they don't get so tired all the time, and that those stairs really aren't so bad. Since these muscles do get worked the hardest regularly, have a little more time between Leg Days than other focus days. They will get extremely sore, especially in the beginning. Push through the first two weeks though, and a little soreness will be something you'll chase after! Per usual, take the time relearn how to do some basic exercises and learn some new ones to add to your routine:

- Squats—Oh, squats. Guaranteed results, guaranteed burn. Here's how to do them properly with your own body weight: Start standing straight with your feet shoulder width apart. Keep back straight and lower yourself solely by bending your knees, stop when thighs are slightly above parallel to the floor. Try to center your weight on your heels, and push back up slowly to the start position. If you're just starting out, don't push yourself past 10 reps, and build slowly.

- Lunges—Works your legs and glutes in a similar way. Ensure when lunging that your body is staying straight and your knees stay off the floor—it's more important to do them slowly and properly than go quickly. Do less reps if you're concerned about time/difficulty.

- Burpees—These are more of a full body workout, but we'll categorize them under legs because that's what ends up working the hardest. If you are lucky enough to have blissfully unaware of burpees before, it's time to get acquainted. Note

33

that this is an extremely challenging exercise, so start off doing as many reps as you feel comfortable. Start in a push up position, complete a push up and then use your upward momentum to spring your legs underneath you. Once you're in a crouch, release and stretch your body up towards the ceiling! Back down to starting position (hop your legs back out), and you've completed your first burpee! Only doing three (or one) is okay until you build your body strength and get the hang of the spastic movements!

- Calf Lifts—All that is required for this quick workout is a surface you can stand on with a few inch dip (think stairs, door ways). Keep the balls of your feet on the very edge of the elevated, and use your calves to lift yourself up and down a few inches. You'll feel the burn faster than you think!

- Stretch your leg muscles every day. Toe touches, quad stretches, really anything that help relieve tension in the most worked part of your body!

Chapter 6

Don't Fall For the Fads

You almost can't make it through a commercial break on network television without seeing an advertisement for one of the many weight loss programs out there, such as Jenny Craig, Weight Watchers or Nutrisystem. There are always ads in our favorite magazines that feature the next new weight loss pill that is guaranteed to work in x days. Fad diets come and go, and every one has wondered if perhaps they too need to cleanse the toxins from their bodies. Now, these fads in nutrition and weight loss aren't all necessarily evil; in fact, the added support of being in such a large group can help ensure you lose the weight you want to lose. However when treading into the waters of popular weight loss solutions, you will need to stay informed and make decisions that are healthy for your body and mind.

Paid Programming (And Eating)

Many people have had success from joining programs like South Beach Diet and Weight Watchers. These programs have benefits, but are costly and not necessary to building a healthier life. These programs do yield results if you follow them to a tee, and offer a large support system to boot. It makes perfect sense why these programs work, because what it all comes down to is counting calories and eating proper portion sizes. These are grounds for any diet, so of course it works. You can accomplish similar meals on your own at a much cheaper price—the Internet has tons of copycat recipes! The convenience and support of these programs makes it almost worth the price.

Don't Eat That

Treat any fad diet with caution. Some examples of popular fad diets of the last two decades: Paleo, Mediterranean, Raw Food, Atkins. Some fad diets may "work", but take a second to notice what all of the fad diets in common: they pretty much all say to cut back on butter, salt, high cholesterol foods—all of the foods you should cut back on when trying to start losing weight anyways. Many these diets cut out a hugely important vitamin or other nutritional requirement, or are just so ludicrously difficult to follow that even the most focused dieter may give up and end up at the bottom of a pint of ice cream.

Give or Take a Little Poison

Supplements and detoxes should be treated with extreme caution. Going a month without alcohol or taking vitamins is one thing, but the trendy pills and 9.5-Day Detox programs can be downright harmful to your health.

If you are unsure as to what a detox is, it's a cleansing of your body for toxins. In theory, this is a good thing! There are toxins your body, but you don't necessarily have to swear of food to get rid of them. There are natural way to promote natural detoxification in your body, such as drinking lemon water in the morning and lightly massaging your muscles. And if there is a type of juice cleanse or detox you would like do for your body to cleanse out the "build up", wait until your body is in physical shape. In summary, do not try to use a detox for weight loss purposes. Furthermore if you are truly wanting to build a healthier lifestyle that will last, avoid flashy diet pills that promise instant weight loss: without diet and exercise, they almost never work (deeming them pointless).

In conclusion, if you want to incorporate any of these trends into your new lifestyle, tread with caution. It's wise to know about these fad diets, but it's even better to pull bits and pieces from different diets (the parts that actually make sense) to find a healthy eating plan that is all your own!

Reap The Benefits of Real Change

Once you've started making the necessary lifestyle changes, you will start to see some benefits right away! You'll find that you can do so much more physically than you ever imagined. Your clothes will fit better and your skin will be clearer, and you'll likely have a little extra pep in your step. Sleep will come easier and you'll feel more alert and focused throughout the day. It's never too late to start and reap all of the benefits that come with living a healthier life!

Maintaining a healthy weight (a by product of proper diet and exercise) can add years to your life. Think about how long you want to be around—do you hope to someday be a great grandparent? Here's some extra motivation if you still needed it: being physically healthy actually prevents diseases including cardiovascular disease, osteoporosis, diabetes, arthritis, and cancer. A healthy weight also helps regulate blood pressure, preventing heart attacks and blood clots. Your immune system will be overall higher than before, keeping you above the common cold!

Not to mention, proper diet and exercise does wonders for a person's headspace and the way they feel about themselves. As the unnecessary pounds shed and clothes become a little looser, you will feel more confident in your skin. The human body *wants* you to be active and eat right, so it makes sure to compensate for it with mood boosting endorphins. Exercise specifically has been linked to helping all sorts of mental health issues, like depression, stress, anxiety, ADHD, and even PTSD. Regularly taking care of your body improves your self worth and empowers you to stay resilient. You'll find that when faced with a crisis, you can handle things better mentally and emotionally. Losing weight is a great goal, but it shouldn't necessarily be the focus. It is more of a great byproduct of a healthier diet and regular exercise.

Conclusion

Thank you for making it through to the end of the end of *Losing Weight: Making a Lifestyle Change*, let's hope it was informative and able to provide you with all of the tools you need to achieve your goals whatever they may be. There is a lot of information (and misinformation) out there about weight loss, and unfortunately so many weight loss plans go array. But now you know that losing weight is a great goal, but it's only a byproduct of the real goal: a healthier life.

The next step is to put your knowledge into application! This book is here to help you from the start of your weight loss journey—from finding motivation to making the ultimate smoothie. Continue to eat conscientiously and workout regularly, and you will find the results you are seeking. Try out some of the recipes found in this book that work great with meal prep and make some of your own smoothie and shake recipes! Always make sure that you are practicing the right way to do common exercises, and keep added some new ones to your repertoire. Start small, stay slow, and never stop believing in yourself (cheesy but true).

Living healthy is a choice, and in this book you learned how to make the right decisions. Your healthy lifestyle plan is unique and you should always continue to tweak it! And don't forget to share your successes with others, so that they may be able to see the same results that you will!

Finally, if you found this book useful in anyway, a review on Amazon is always appreciated!

Made in the USA
Middletown, DE
12 May 2017

43572759R00027